T0128900

Food and Water

Food and Water

Aung Chin Win Aung

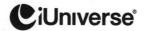

FOOD AND WATER

iUniverse books may be ordered through booksellers or by contacting:

iUniverse
1663 Liberty Drive
Bloomington, IN 47403
www.iuniverse.com
1-800-Authors (1-800-288-4677)

ISBN: 978-1-5320-7304-5 (sc)
ISBN: 978-1-5320-7305-2 (e)

Print information available on the last page.

iUniverse rev. date: 04/09/2019

Introduction

This book is about food and water including air but most of the presentations are humans and animals. Humans kill animals for food, for money and for fun. This book tells of how humans and animals survive. They eat food and drink water as well as air they breathe. When looking at the situation of human population, the planet is big enough for consumption of natural resources. Birds in the air, fishes in the water, and animals on the land are disappeared by human cruelties.

Leo Taylor

Author Aung Chin Win Aung
Reference
History of the earth
History of Universe
Indian Philosophy
Greek Philosophy
Relationships between animals and humans
Living creatures on earth
Animal and Human life
Milky Way and glacier
Animal and human civilization
Ancient ancestors

Slaughtering and killing of animals are not fun. Most hunters think killing of animals is fun and spot. If they care of animal-suffering including themselves might get some lessons.

Humans are the most dangerous creature on earth. They have killed their own creature than any other animals on earth. They destroyed more ecosystems than any other animals. They have made species extinct more than any other animals. Unlike any other animals on earth human has created different weapons that kill more living creatures. No animal on earth other than human beings have created bombs, poisonous chemicals, bio-toxins, cars, planes, heavy machinery and all other things that kill all living creatures and destroy environment directly or indirectly. Thinking of a dangerous animal about how physically powerful it is and how savage it can be but human-brain is smarter than any other animals. The most interesting thing is how humans use technology to change the globe. Animals used to be tools for human beings and they are used for farming and other laborers but when technology changed the globe, animals become free from labors exact for food. It is sad. Human beings are not animals but creatures. However, what makes human beings more dangerous than any other animals or any other creatures that hurt people because of their own ego while animals on the other hand instinctively kill to fulfill their desire. It is known that the lion is the king of the jungle because of strength and power as well as ability to kill any creature including humans. It is always remarkable to see an animal overcome such a creature however, like any other animal it relies on instinct and is concerned with fulfilling the desire.

It is a reasoning mind that makes humans so dangerous. The reasoning mind lets people understand and manipulate reality for their own ends. In the Stone Age, humans became powerful and dangerous to mammoths. Since then, the knowledge and technology have grown immensely and humans now rule the planet and between guns and bombs, nothing can match for danger.

Humans kill other creatures and humans other than hunger and survival. Humans are meant to the world-deadliest animal other than any animals. While the historians search through the history it shows a list of animals such as alligators, sharks, wolfs, tigers and lions are the most dangerous animals in the world. But humans kill those deadliest animals for skin some for their tusks and so on, according to a survey on intentional homicide almost half million peoples have lost their lives. Actually, animals do not attack the others unless they are hungry. They do not kill other animals including humans for fun. People label this or that animal as the most dangerous, depending on whether they want to travel, Africa, Sweden, Australia and Asia as well as other continents.

What context would be pushing forward if animals were to label the human as the most dangerous animal?

Mankind has developed technology far beyond anything any other animals. Mankind has directly and indirectly driven to extinction far more other animal species than any other animals and mankind has killed more of their own species than any other animals. Mankind is far more dangerous than any other animal species alive or extinct. Homo sapiens do not superficially fit the world's most dangerous animal, but appearances are very deceptive. Homo could not built weapons, like fangs, talons, claws, horns, and tusks. Homo is very slow, does not climb or swim very well, and cannot fly. Homo sapiens have hands with opposable thumbs, and an advanced brain to use them for the creation of dead.

Tigers may be strong with sharp teeth. Bears may be super strong with big claws. Alligators have the ability to tear entire limbs off. But nothing beats a human with a machine gun. Humans also destroy the environment, farm animals for food, build nuclear weapons, and they love to have war with nation states. Why humans are dangerous to earth is a longer debate. Human overtime has proved that natural environment could be damaged by human species than any other creatures. Animals do not create deadly weapons to destroy planet. Human beings are certainly the most vicious and bloodthirsty.

Halal is killing of animals in Islamic idea that permissible to slaughter animals for people gatherings as well as religious activities. The people who kill animals for people gathering and religious activities do not care of animal-suffering. The suffering of living creatures is the Jewish principle that bans on pain on animals. This concept is not clearly enunciated in the written Torah, but accepted by the Talmud as being a biblical mandate.

The Humane Slaughter Act is the United States federal law formulated to decrease livestock suffering during slaughter. The act was approved on August 27, 1958. Animals kill animals for food are considered instinct. There are several dangerous animals in the water and land. In the water the largest killer is the blue whale that is considered a largest animal on earth. But the blue whale is killed by human. Chimpanzees wage war against rival groups, killing rival males and eating the baby chimps. Animals also wage warfare on other animals like human beings. Many insects like ants are waging war on other ants and engaging cannibalism. Also many plants are dangerous to animals and humans. Eating a dangerous plant can cause seizures, spasms, tremors, gastroenteritis, cardiovascular collapse, coma, and then death. Many plants kill animals by trapping or poisoning them, then digesting them for nourishment. Some plants kill rodent with various methods.

In North America, hunters use deadly weapons to kill bear, wolf, caribou, moose, sheep and bison. In South America, dear and other species are hunted. In Asia, several species of animals like deer, bear, sheep, tiger and other animals are hunted. In Australia, deer and wild boar are hunted. Hunting game, small or big, is to kill animals for food, meat, horn, bone, trophy or spot. The term is historically associated with the hunting of Africa-hunting, lion, African elephant, Cape buffalo, leopard and rhinoceros, and with tigers and rhinoceroses, on the Indian subcontinent. The hunting, along with the big five animals, many other species like kudu, antelope, and hartebeest. Moose, elk, bear, mountain lion, caribou, bison and deer are the largest game hunted in North America, which is where most big-game hunting is conducted. Big-game hunting is conducted in Africa, North America, South America, Europe, Asia and Australia. In Africa, lion, Cape buffalo, elephant, giraffe and other large game animals are hunted. Many species of animals are disappeared because of hunting games in the world.

People for the Ethical Treatment of Animals (PETA) are an animal rights group founded in America and is based in Norfolk, Virginia. It is led by Ingrid Newkirk, it claims to have million members and supporters, which would make it the largest animal rights group in the world. The slogan is animals are not to eat, wear, experiment, entertainment, or abuse in any other way. Veganism is the practice of abstaining from the use of all animal products, particularly in diet.

Human is the most cruel and dangerous creature to the animals and the world. Human entertainment is animal to fight each other like dog fight, cock fight, bull fight and many other animals including insects.

Vegetarianism is the practice of abstaining from the consumption of meat, red meat, poultry, seafood, insects and the flesh of any other animal and may also include abstention from by-products of animal slaughter. Vegetarians, however, may consume eggs, dairy products and honey. Ahimsa is an important tenet of 3 religions, Jainism, Hinduism, and Buddhism. Ahimsa is a multidimensional concept, inspired by the premise that all living beings have the spark of the spiritual energy;

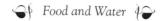

therefore, to hurt another being is to hurt one-self. Ahimsa has also been related to the notion that any violence has karmic consequences.

Scientists revealed millions of years ago, several species of human-like creatures wandered around the landscape of wilderness. Some looked surprisingly similar to each other, while others had distinct, defining features. Hundreds of bones discovered in a cave are now believed to be a new species, known as Homo Naledi. There may be many more extinct Hominin species. Modern species appeared around 200,000 years ago, at a time when several others existed.

Human-like species-known as Hominins-died out and one species of human, the great apes, and other six species, chimpanzees, bonobos, two species of gorilla and two species of orangutan. There are some clues that reveal why some of ancestors were more successful than others. Several million years ago, when a great many Hominin species lived side-by-side, they mainly ate plants. There is no evidence they were systematically preying on large animals. They may have been wiped out by a large volcanic eruption, according to geological evidence from the area. Living on one small island would also leave a species more vulnerable to extinction when natural disaster strikes. People do not know enough about the (Denisova Hominins) that are an extinct species or subspecies of archaic human in the genus Homo. People came to know a lot more about the Neanderthals after studying about human beings.

Why were the only human species left behind and why did they die out and the temperature did not have anything to do with main problem?

The climate seemed to change the environment they lived in, and they did not adapt their hunting style for survival. Neanderthals were better adapted to hunting in woodland atmospheres than modern humans. But when European climate began fluctuating, the forests became more open, becoming more like the African savannahs that modern humans were used to. The forests provided most of Neanderthals to have foods, but later dwindled and could no longer sustain them. Modern humans also seemed to hunt a greater range of species. They also hunted smaller animals like hares and rabbits.

There is little evidence that Neanderthals hunted similar small ground mammals according to analyses of archaeological sites where the Neanderthals clung on the longest. The weapons they made were better appropriate for hunting larger animals. The evidence revealed that they ate birds and they may have lured them in with the remains of other dead animal carcasses, rather than actively hunting them in the sky. But tools are not the only things modern humans made. They created other things too.

There was sufficient evidence that they were making art. Archaeologists have found ornaments, jewelry, figurative depictions of mythical animals and even musical instruments. They made a lot of wooden carvings of animal figures like a lion-human statue and many others found in a cave. Similar sculptures were found elsewhere in Europe. Symbols were a kind of social connection. They could help people organize their social and economic affairs with one another. Neanderthals did not seem to need art or symbols. There was limited evidence they made some jewelry, but not to the extent. Hunting, cooking, sleeping, eating, sex and recreation were their occupations.

Evolutionary theory seemed to be more complicated. Homo erectus survived for a long time and was the first Hominin species to expand out of Africa before even the Neanderthals but its brain was not big enough to do what they wanted to. Some anthropologists were uncomfortable with the idea that big brains were the solution. Big brains may have played a role in success, but Neanderthals had equally large brains compared to their body size. Most Europeans developed a tolerance to lactose when the ancestors started to eat more dairy produce. Genetic changes can also occur when large populations are faced with devastating diseases such as the Black Death in the 14th Century, which changed the genes of survivors. 100,000 years of existence, modern humans behaved much like Neanderthals.

Researchers agreed that ancient ancestors, the upright walking apes, ascended in Africa. But the discovery of a new primate that lived about 37 million years ago in the ancient swamplands of Asia supports the idea that the primate family that gave rise to humans was rooted in Asia. The discovery suggested that the ancestors of all monkeys, apes, and humans-known as the anthropoids-arose in Asia and made the arduous journey to the island continent of Africa almost 40 million years ago. The fossils of anthropoid were found in North Africa and dated to about 30 million years ago. Researchers introduced discovering the remains of petite primates that lived 37 million to 45 million years ago in China, Burma, and other Asian nations. This suggested that anthropoids may have actually arisen in Asia and then migrated to Africa a few million years later. But paleontologists lacked the fossils to show when and how these anthropoids trekked from Asia to Africa. How did they travel from Asia to Africa was unknown. An international team of researchers excavated the fossils of early fish, turtle, and ancestral hippo teeth from fossil beds near the village of Nyaungpinle in Burma found a molar the size of a kernel of popcorn. The tooth, dated to about 38 million years ago, belonged to a new species of ancient primate. It was the size of a small chipmunk. After several more years of arduous fieldwork, the team collected just four molars of this primitive anthropoid because it was a difficult place to work and it took many years to find teeth. When the researchers examined the teeth from the two primates under a microscope, they were so similar in size, shape, and age that they could have belonged to the same species of primate. The team noticed that the new molars from the Asian Afrasia (Afro-Eurasia) were more primitive than those of Afrotarsius (primate) from Libya, particularly in the larger size of a tiny bulge at the back of its last lower molar. These primitive traits, as well as the greater diversity and age of early or stem anthropoids in Asia rather than Africa suggest that this group arose in Asia and migrated to Africa 37 million to 39 million years ago.

Out-of-Asia seemed to be convoluted. The team proposed that more than one species of anthropoid migrated from Asia to Africa at the time, because there were at least two other types of early anthropoids alive at about the same time as Afrotarsius in Libya; but they were not closely related to Afrotarsius or Afrasia. Others agreed that if both the new species of primates from Burma and Libya are indeed early anthropoids, they would greatly strengthen the case for the Asian origins of anthropoids. It would show that there was a major migration of primates and probably other mammals between the two continents at a time when it was not easy to get across the ancient ocean that divided Africa from Asia. The deepest primate roots were in Asia, not Africa.

The Greek Philosopher presented the four elements, earth, water, air and fire for civilizations. The civilizations were proposed to explain the nature and complexity of all matter in terms of simpler substances. Ancient cultures in Babylonia, Japan, Tibet and India had similar views and they sometimes refer to local languages "air" as "wind" and the fifth element as "void". The idea of East and West is similar because of the view of the cosmological elements. These different cultures and even individual philosophers had widely varying explanations concerning their attributes and how they related to observable phenomena as well as cosmology. Sometimes these theories covered with mythology and were personified in deities. Some of these interpretations included atomism (the idea of very small, indivisible portions of matter) but other interpretations considered the elements to be divisible into infinitely small pieces without changing their nature. While the classification of the material world in ancient civilization like Indian Hellenistic Egypt and ancient Greece, Air, Earth, Fire and Water, was more philosophical. Medieval Middle Eastern scientists used practical, experimental observation to classify materials. In Europe, the Ancient Greek philosopher Aristotle-system evolved slightly into the medieval system and for the first time in Europe that became subject to experimental verification in the 1600s, during the Scientific Revolution. Modern science does not support the classical elements as the material basis of the physical world. Atomic theory classifies atoms into more than a hundred chemical elements such as oxygen, iron and mercury. These elements form chemical compounds and mixtures, and under different temperatures and pressures, these substances can adopt different state of matter. The most commonly observed states of solid, liquid, gas, and plasma share many attributes with the classical elements of earth, water, air, and fire, respectively, but these states are due to similar behavior of different types of atoms at similar energy levels, and not due to containing a certain type of atom or a certain type of substance. In classical thought, the four elements, earth, water, air, fire as proposed by Empedocles frequently occur; Aristotle added a fifth element, aether, it has been called Akasha (space) in India and quintessence in Europe.

The concept of the five elements formed a basis of analysis in ancient civilization, particularly in an esoteric context, the four states-of-matter describe matter, and a fifth element describes that was beyond the material world. Similar lists existed in ancient Asian civilization. The four great elements, and two others sometimes added, are not viewed as substances, but as categories of sensory experience.

In Babylonian mythology, the cosmogony was written between the 18th and 16th centuries BC, as personified cosmic elements: sea, earth, sky, and wind. In other Babylonian texts these phenomena are considered independent of their association with deities, though they were not treated as the component elements of the universe, as later in Empedocles.

The system of five elements was found in Indian Civilization or the five great elements. The suggested was that all of formation, including the human body made up of these five essential elements and that upon death, the human body dissolves into these five elements of nature and balance the natural cycle.

The five elements are associated with the five senses, and act as the gross medium for the experience of sensations. The basest element, earth, using all the other elements, can be perceived by all five senses, hearing, touch, sight, taste, and smell. The next higher element, water, has no odor but can be heard, felt, seen and tasted. Fire can be heard, felt and seen. Air can be heard and felt. "Akasha" (aether) is beyond the senses of smell, taste, sight, and touch; it is being accessible to the sense of hearing alone.

In the great elements or four elements are earth, water, fire and air. The four elements are a basis for understanding of suffering and for liberating oneself from suffering. The earliest civilizations explained that the four primary material elements are the sensory qualities, solidity, fluidity, temperature, and mobility; their characterization as earth, water, fire, and air, respectively, is declared an abstraction-instead of concentrating on the fact of material existence, one observes how a physical thing is sensed, felt, perceived.

The teaching regarding the four elements is to be understood as the base of all observation of real sensations rather than as a philosophy. The four properties are cohesion (water), solidity or inertia (earth), expansion or vibration (air) and heat or energy content (fire). It promulgated a categorization of mind and matter as composed of the four elements.

Just as a skilled butcher or his apprentice, having killed a cow, would sit at a crossroads cutting it up into pieces, the religious person anticipates the body and stands as well as it is disposed: The religious person claim every part of the body as the earth property, liquid property, fire property and wind property. The pain of the suffering is mind and matter.

The Chinese had a somewhat different series of elements, namely Fire, Earth, Metal (literally gold), Water and Wood, which were understood as different types of energy in a state of constant interaction and flux with one another, rather than the Western notion of different kinds of material.

Although it is usually translated as "element", the Chinese literally means something like changing states of being "permutations" or "metamorphoses of being". In fact sinologist (Chinese language) cannot agree on any single translation. The Chinese elements were seen as ever changing and moving one translation of the five changes.

An ancient mnemonic device is used for systems with five stages; hence the translation of "movements", "phases" or "steps" over "elements." is preferred.

In Chinese text the universe consists of heaven and earth. The five major planets are associated with and even named after the elements: Jupiter is Wood, Mars is Fire, Saturn is Earth, Venus is Metal and Mercury is Water. The Moon represents Yin, and the Sun represents Yang. Yin, Yang, and the five elements are associated with themes in the oldest Chinese classical transcripts which describes an ancient system of cosmology and philosophy. The five elements also play an important part in Chinese philosophy. The Chinese form the geomancy known as Feng shui (wind-water).

The doctrine of five segments describes two cycles of balance, a generating or formation cycle and an overcoming or destruction cycle of interactions between the phases. There are also two cycles of imbalance, an overacting cycle and an insulting cycle.

The ancient Greek belief in five basic elements, earth, water, air, fire and aether, dates from pre-Socratic times and persisted throughout the Middle Ages and into the Renaissance deeply influencing European notion and culture.

Extracted from Greek philosophy, Indian philosophy and Wikipedia

NOTES:

NOTES:

NOTES:

NOTES:

NOTES:

NOTES:

NOTES:

NOTES:

NOTES:

NOTES:

NOTES:

NOTES:

NOTES:

NOTES:

NOTES:

NOTES:

NOTES:

NOTES:

NOTES:

NOTES:

NOTES:

NOTES:

NOTES:

NOTES:

NOTES:

NOTES:

NOTES:

NOTES:

NOTES:

NOTES:

NOTES:

NOTES:

NOTES:

NOTES:

NOTES:

NOTES:

NOTES:

NOTES:

NOTES:

NOTES:

NOTES:

Printed in the United States
By Bookmasters